Breakthrough to Weight Loss Success

David Shipp

"Get your head in the right place for weight loss success"

First published in Great Britain 2010

Second edition published in Great Britain in 2011-01-28

ShippShape
david@shippshape.com
www.shippshape.com

ISBN 978-1-4461-2380-5

CONTENTS

Introduction

The theory of losing weight is simple. Putting this theory into practice is a challenge met by thousands of people around the world each and everyday. You probably already know how to lose weight, but what is it that stops you from achieving your weight loss goals and more importantly maintaining the weight you wish to be?

There is no shortage of diets, pills and products promising quick and easy weight loss, many of them have the potential to work, but have they worked for **you**? The majority of approaches to losing weight fail to address the real reasons why weight was gained in the first place.

The reasons why someone over-eats or gives into temptation are rarely addressed and resolved. Someone can logically know that eating lots of chocolate bars is not going to support their goal of weight loss, but due to some reason they still consume them. From my experience, most people know what they need to do to lose weight. The biggest challenge people face is keeping their motivation going and not falling into bad habits. I continually hear people say they know they could lose weight if only they were in the 'right frame of mind'. Is this something you say?

There is an abundance of information on '**how-to**' do anything we wish, but the real challenge is putting this knowledge into action. You may want to lose weight and know how to do it, but if you are reading this book, my guess is you have struggled to achieve your goal up to now. To be able to put the knowledge into action relies on two things. You must have the correct information and you must understand why you and your body behave the way they do. This book will address both topics.

By reading this book you will discover how the processes of gaining, maintaining and losing weight are all related to the automatic behaviours of your physical body. If you want to achieve any of these results, it is important to know what goes on inside your body.

You will also discover and look to resolve the reasons why you might over-eat or lose motivation.

Armed with the knowledge of the physical and psychological aspects you will be in a much better position to achieve permanent weight loss success.

A frustration of mine with regards to the weight loss industry is the promise of a quick fix. With the exception of liposuction where you physically remove weight from the body, weight loss will take a certain amount of time. Gaining weight takes time; losing weight will also take time.

Time is obviously a key issue for anyone wanting to lose weight, as they want results straight away. I can appreciate this, but the use of many pills, products and eating plans on the market just cannot be sustained. Although they may get results in the short term they do not address and resolve the real reason why weight was gained in the first place. You can still over-eat and give into temptation while on a diet. We must ascend above the fad diets and the so-called magic pills and concentrate on the facts.

The emphasis of this book is on helping you get in the correct frame of mind. To do this we will be studying human behaviour on many levels. We will clarify how the physical body behaves with regards to gaining and losing weight. We will also look at the behaviour of eating and drinking and how this obviously has a large impact on weight loss. From understanding the fundamentals of human behaviour you will discover what aspects are under your control, and accept those that are not.

It doesn't matter how long weight has been a problem, you will learn from this book that the reason you have not lost the weight is actually down to your psychology and behaviour more than anything else. You will be pleased to know that whatever the problem may be, it can be resolved and by reading this book you have taken a very important step.

I learnt a long time ago that I will never know enough about anyone else to fully understand what life is like for them. This is the underlying theme throughout this whole book. In every sense of the word you are unique. You have unique feelings, thoughts, opinions, memories and so on. The reason why one person over-eats or avoids exercise will not necessarily be the same for someone else. No one sees, hears, feels exactly what you feel, you have an exclusive interpretation of the world, by simply being you. Because of this, I have tried to speak directly to you as the reader, and offer you a unique experience of what you are about to read. What is more important than the words I write is what you believe and take in.

A great example of this individuality is the well known question 'does my bum look big in this?' Whether you have asked your spouse this question doesn't matter. What does matter is whether you would believe them whatever answer they gave. Think about this for a moment. You probably asked the question because you feel that your bum does look big. If your spouse answered 'no', would it put your mind at ease or would you still think and feel that your bum looks big?

It is never what happens in life that matters, its how you perceive it. This book is about your unique situation and taking steps to improve it for the better. I cannot emphasis enough how important it is for you to read this book in relation to yourself.

I hope to meet you at a ShippShape event soon!

David Shipp

CHAPTER 1

A STORY OF SURVIVAL

When did weight loss become so confusing? There are thousands of diets and approaches to weight loss, but I am going to keep it simple and talk about the human body rather than an 'approach' or 'theory'. Gaining, maintaining and losing weight is an energy balance within the human body.

In simple terms if you consume more energy (calories in food and drink) than the body uses, the excess energy will be stored as fat in tissue around the body. Likewise, if the body is not receiving the energy it requires through food and drink, then the body will use the energy stored as fat to make up the shortfall. I appreciate that this is a very simple description of how the body gains and loses weight physically, but most **healthy** diets and weight loss programmes are based on these facts, and if followed will bring about results.

It all sounds so simple; to lose weight you must cut down on the energy going into the body, and/or use up more energy through exercise or daily activities. Out of the two options, research has shown that the easiest and quickest way to get weight loss results is to cut down on the energy going into the body. The simple reason is that you can eat/consume calories quicker than you can use them up in a specific period of time. For example, you could eat 200 calories in two minutes (two chocolate bars), but you would have to jog for thirty minutes to burn off the same amount of calories. This is not to say exercise is not important. There are many physical and psychological benefits brought about from physical activity including enhanced weight loss. Because eating and the calorie consumption side of the energy balance has the most impact on weight loss, this is where we are going to concentrate our efforts.

In the following chapters we will discuss how the physical body behaves with regards to gaining, maintaining and losing weight. I highlighted in the introduction of this book, that having the correct information is of utmost importance if you want to turn knowledge into action and achieve weight loss success.

I'm sure you will agree that the human body is a very complex organism. I cannot discuss every little detail about the physical body, but we will be looking at the primary parts and systems in the body that relate to the gain and loss of weight. The examples I have used highlight how the body reacts in different scenarios and will answer questions you may have had about some of the approaches to weight loss that have been recommended in the past.

Hopefully by the end of this book you will begin to appreciate how everything in the body is connected in some way or form. What we see and experience is only the tip of the iceberg of what is actually happening inside the body.

Before concentrating specifically on weight, we must look at the big picture of what your body does. We can then start to understand the real reasons why we behave the way we do, physically and psychologically, with regards to gaining, maintaining and losing weight.

I do not have an answer for why we have a body and why there is life on earth, but it is clear that at some time in the past, life began. From looking at the history of the human body it is clear that although our environments and lifestyles have changed over countless years, in essence the way we function, physically and psychologically is no different. The big picture of what your body does is defined by a single word: survival. Please commit this to memory as it has the power to explain everything we do both physically and psychologically.

You will learn from this book that the reason we are able to survive is due to many different actions. Collectively they can be described as the ability to adapt to our surroundings at any moment in time. Why we have the ability to survive and what we are surviving for are once again questions I cannot answer, but it is clear that survival is our highest priority. It is mesmerizing the work your physical body does, much of which happens automatically.

This book is not the place for me to describe in detail every function of the body, but please appreciate that everything your body does automatically points to one subject; survival. As you continue to read, you will discover more and more that the drive to survive explains everything we do in every part of our lives. If you are not convinced, and wondering what this all has to do with losing weight, keep an open mind and please read on.

CHAPTER 2

THE ABILITY TO ADAPT

Before we go any further we must continue to discuss the big picture of what the body does and look at why we are able to survive. The information in this chapter is not necessarily weight loss specific but is important in understanding where weight gain and loss begins.

As I have said in the previous chapter we will be concentrating on your eating behaviours, as this has the most impact on weight loss and is often the biggest challenge for people wanting to lose weight. The information in this chapter will also be relevant when we later discuss the importance of your psychology with regards to weight loss. Our survival relies on many aspects but they can all be summed up by our ability to adapt to our immediate environment at any given point in time. Our ability to adapt can explain every behaviour that we perform, both on a physical and psychological level.

Whatever is happening in your immediate surroundings, everything is continuously changing on a second-to-second basis. It has changed throughout your life depending on what you see, hear, touch, taste, smell, where you are and the experiences you are having. Also on a second-to-second basis, your body is making sure that life is being sustained. If there is a threat to survival, the body will do what it can and adapt to the situation at hand. We will be looking closely at this important system of sensing and reacting. It is happening in every area of your life and answers the question why we are able to survive.

We will begin by looking at an automatic behaviour familiar to everyone. If you are exposed to extreme temperatures your body will react accordingly. If your body is exposed to warm temperatures you will sweat or perspire. This reaction is an effort to cool down vital parts of the physical body. By releasing water on to the surface of the skin, the fluid will evaporate allowing the body to cool. Your skin will also turn red due to an increase of blood rushing towards the outside the body away from vital organs that are susceptible to overheating. Your body will sense that you are losing fluid through sweat and send signals to the brain to consume more water.

The opposite is also true when we are exposed to cold temperatures. The outside of the body will become pale as blood rushes towards the vital organs to keep them warm and working.

We will be inclined to seek shelter and warmth. Goosebumps will raise the hair on your body to provide more insulation between the skin and the cold air. Shivering tightens the skin and shakes the muscles in an attempt to conserve and generate heat to warm the body up.

In the above example, the body knows what temperature is best to sustain life without any problems. We know this temperature is approximately 37 degrees Celsius, but the body automatically concentrates its efforts on keeping it at this value. If there is a threat of the temperature changing, the body will take whatever action it has to. The balance or homeostasis the body is seeking is a very important concept to remember. It shows that your body knows what is needed and automatically behaves in a way that is suitable.

The above example can also demonstrate the versatility of the human body to adapt. Continued exposure to heat or cold can result in what we know as acclimatization. We know that if we are exposed to certain temperatures for a period of time we can get 'used' to it. Being exposed to excessive temperatures for a period of time can bring about physiological changes including more active sweating in response to continued heat and an increase in fat deposits in response to continued cold.

It is important to understand how your body reacts to the outside environment and can automatically sense threats to your survival. The different parts that make up the nervous system are the primary ways in which we make meaning of our surrounding environment and then initiate reactions in appropriate parts of the body in order to survive.

The nervous system is a network of specialised cells that process and transfer important signals and impulses throughout the body. It is made up of the central nervous system (CNS) and the peripheral nervous system (PNS). The central nervous system involves the brain and the spinal cord. The CNS coordinates the activity of all the parts of the body; it is devoted to processing information and together with the PNS has a fundamental role in the control of behaviour.

The PNS is the link between the central nervous system and the body's organs and limbs. The PNS is also split into two parts, the somatic nervous system (SNS) and the autonomic nervous system (ANS). The SNS is associated with the processing of information from external stimuli, through receptors connected to sense organs. This is important to survival because it helps the body keep in touch with its surroundings.

The sense organs involved are not limited to sight (eyes), hearing (ears), touch (skin), taste (taste buds) and smell (nose). The SNS is also concerned with the sense of temperature (as in our example), balance, acceleration, position of body and pain. Pain signals that there is damage to tissue whether it is inside or on the outside of the body. Pain can be felt through the touch of something hot, but can equally be felt if we have a sore knee and is within the body itself.

The SNS is responsible for coordinating voluntary body movements through the action of skeletal muscles. Skeletal muscle is one of the three major types of muscle, the others being cardiac and smooth. Skeletal muscle is used to move the body and can be finely controlled. This type of muscle can range from your bicep to the small muscles that control eye movements. It is 'voluntary muscle', which means we are aware of these types of muscle in use.

Out of all the parts of the nervous system, the autonomic nervous system (ANS) is particularly important to survival. The ANS acts as a control system, which maintains the homeostasis of the human body. Homeostasis is simply the human body's ability to regulate its inner environment, to ensure its stability in response to fluctuations in the outside environment. The ANS affects heart rate, digestion, metabolism, respiration rate, salivation, perspiration, diameter of pupils, urination and sexual arousal. Most of the actions are involuntary and happen without us knowing anything about them.

The autonomic nervous system is responsible for carrying signals and impulses to three types of human tissue; these are cardiac muscle, smooth muscle and glandular tissue. Cardiac muscle is found in the heart and is involuntary; we all take it for granted that these muscles continuously propel blood around the body to keep us alive. Smooth muscle is also an involuntary type of muscle. It is found within other organ systems and internal functions of the body. An example of this type of muscle is the muscles that move food through the process of digestion. Glandular tissue is primarily involved in the release of hormones within the body and bodily fluids outside the body including sweat. Hormones are basically chemicals released by one or more cells that have the ability to affect other cells and parts of the body. We will return to speak about hormones throughout this book as they have a considerable impact on your behaviour physically and psychologically.

The autonomic nervous system is made up of the sympathetic system (SS) and the parasympathetic system (PS). The effect on the cardiac muscle, smooth muscle and glandular tissue depends on what level of sympathetic or parasympathetic action is required for homeostasis to occur. In the event our central nervous system perceives we are in danger or stress, the SS will automatically respond, it will cause changes within the body to react to the environment we are in.

The SS is responsible for an individual's acceleration in heart function (cardiac muscle), dilation of pupils (smooth muscle) and the release of the hormone cortisol from the adrenal gland (glandular tissue), to increase blood pressure and blood glucose. Blood glucose will be discussed further in a later chapter. There are many other physiological changes, but this gives you an appreciation how the body gets primed for action and all stems from the central nervous system (brain) perceiving a threat to survival. These actions are collectively known as the fight-or-flight or stress response. It is referred to fight-or-flight, because body is getting ready to do either of these things. In any situation deemed stressful or dangerous, we can either stand up to it or 'run' from it.

The parasympathetic nervous system (PS) in contrast is often referred to as the rest-and-digest response. The PS is evident when a person is in a state of rest or relaxation. It is concerned with the slowing of the heart (cardiac muscle) and the constriction of pupils (smooth muscle). With regard to glandular tissue, the PS is also responsible for stimulating the digestive system to take in food, digest it, extract nutrients and energy, make and repair new cells and expel the remaining waste. As with the SS, there are many other physiological changes that occur.

There is always a balance of both the sympathetic and parasympathetic systems. It is not the case that one is working and the other is having time off. Your body is continually repairing itself, but it will be dependant on your surroundings to what degree. Survival and homeostasis is the goal of the human body.

It is important to remember that the central nervous system (the brain and the spinal cord) controls the body and decides what behaviours happen inside and outside the body. In the following chapter we will look at the system within the body that processes the food you eat and obviously has a large impact on you gaining, maintaining and losing weight.

CHAPTER 3

THE DIGESTIVE SYSTEM

With the topic of survival in mind, we will be looking closely at the systems within the body, which have the most impact on how weight is gained, maintained and lost. With this knowledge you will be in a better position to know how to lose weight physically. The most influential process within the body with regards to physical weight is the digestive system. The digestive system is familiar to all of us as human beings, without it, we would not be alive.

As was discussed in the previous chapter, the digestive system and how well it works is influenced by your surroundings and our stress response. To reiterate, if the senses and the central nervous system (brain and spinal cord) perceive danger, or a threat to survival, the body will focus its attention on activities within the body, which can increase the likelihood of survival. Blood and energy is taken away from parts of the digestive system and as a result, appetite may be lost and the body may not absorb nutrients that are available in the food you have actually eaten. Throughout this chapter I will concentrate on how the digestive system functions if there was no immediate threat to survival.

Without food there is only so long you can survive. All food must go through the complex process of being broken down into the nutrients that cells can use to build and operate their parts. Each bite of food must first be reduced into smaller pieces by the teeth. These pieces can then be further broken down by enzymes in saliva and other body chemicals to yield glucose, the amino acids of proteins, the simple sugars of carbohydrates, the acids that make up fats and oils and the nucleic acids that make up DNA. After the small pieces of food are swallowed and pass down the oesophagus (food pipe), the body automatically continues the work of digesting the food you have just eaten.

The food then enters the stomach where it is stored and mechanically mixed with more enzymes to digest proteins and carbohydrates. A valve at the bottom of the stomach will then let small amounts of partially digested food, called chyme, into the small intestine where most of the absorption of food occurs. The resulting material is so small that it can pass into the tiniest blood vessels to then nourish trillions of cells within the body.

At the same time the partially digested food (chyme) enters the small intestine, three other organs are at work, the pancreas, liver and gall bladder. Their primary function is to release further enzymes into the small intestine so further nutrients can be extracted from the food. After the small intestine, the food passes into the large intestine, often referred to as the colon. The colon's primary function is to absorb water and electrolytes and eliminate solid wastes that the body cannot use through the anus. Electrolytes are chemical salts that nerves and muscles require to function properly.

From the outline above, we can start to look closely at the specific parts of the digestive system. The first important aspect to discuss is what controls the digestive system. What causes saliva and other enzymes to be released and so on. The answer to these questions is the central nervous system and its associated parts. We started our initial description of the digestive system at the moment food was in the mouth, but we could also discuss behaviours prior to this.

In the previous chapter I described the different parts of the nervous system. With so many abbreviations (CNS, PNS, ANS, SNS, PS and SS), you may have been a little confused and I apologise if this was the case. In this part we will also be discussing the nervous system, but I will be describing the behaviours rather than the actually names of the parts that undertake them. Remember that the central nervous system coordinates the activity of all the parts of the body and is devoted to processing information to carry out behaviours. The central nervous system relies on a network of specialised cells, for now we will call nerve cells. Another way the central nervous system controls and adjusts body functions is through the use of hormones released by glands.

There is a major difference between nerve cells and hormones. Nerve cells will travel along nerve pathways to and from the central nervous system, whereas hormones are released into the blood stream and although stimulated by the central nervous system will act on other cells of the body when required. Hormones are among the most abundant and influential chemicals in the body.

As has been stated, we need food to survive. Where the initial stimulus for food comes from is unclear, but it is combination of hormones and nerve cells from different parts of the body. The following is an example of what hormone and nerve behaviours happen in relation to the digestive system.

The stomach and small intestine release the 'hunger' hormone ghrelin in to the blood stream. The hormone reaches receptors in the brain, which coordinates our senses (sight, sound, touch, smell and taste) and our muscles and limbs to seek food.

At the same time, the brain primes the body to receive food, by starting muscle contractions within the digestive system. When food is eaten, it is sensed by the central nervous system. The brain stimulates other glandular tissue including the thyroid to release further hormones into blood stream, which aid digestion and above all the survival of the physical body.

Once the body has had enough food the 'satiety' or 'satisfaction' hormone leptin, is released by the body. Leptin stimulates the brain to suppress appetite and the desire for food. As you can see the central nervous system does a tremendous amount of work. It is not only helping the body adapt to what is going on outside the body, but also what is happening inside to keep the body alive and functioning.

As we discussed earlier the resultant material from digested food is so small it can pass into the tiniest blood vessels and go on to nourish trillions of cells around the body. This minute material from digested food is made up of amino, fatty and nucleic acids, and also glucose. The material enters the blood stream and is transported around the body to help cells repair themselves and create useful energy for the body. The creation of energy within cells and the associated chemical reactions are referred to metabolism.

Metabolism can also be referred to as the amount of energy (calories) your body burns to maintain itself. Whether you are eating, drinking, sleeping, cleaning etc... your body is constantly burning calories to keep you going. All living organisms 'have' a metabolism to harvest energy from organic matter (food) to keep the body working. The glucose and oxygen within the blood stream combine to create energy inside cells, which is the process that provides 'life' in our bodies. Amino, fatty and nucleic acids help the process of metabolism and are required to maintain the cells themselves.

The thyroid gland, which was mentioned earlier, stimulates and regulates your metabolism. The hormone released by the gland can affect every single cell in your body and how much energy is being generated. If there is a threat to survival or a demand for lots of energy, the thyroid will 'speed up' your metabolism. This is a significant behaviour with regards to our stress response discussed in the previous chapter. At times of rest or minimal demand for energy, your metabolism is slower. Therefore, not as much energy is required. Without the thyroid, virtually no major body system can function properly. Once again, recognise how important our immediate surroundings are in relation to the activity of the thyroid. Your surroundings stimulate your nervous system, which in turn stimulates the thyroid gland and its level of activity.

Glucose is the physical body's fuel. It is what every cell in your body uses to do its specific job. Cells are the smallest units of life, so tiny that they are only visible under a microscope. Everything within the physical body is made up of these cells and as you can imagine their importance is paramount. If they are not supplied with enough energy, the cells, and the organs, muscles, tissues etc... they make up will fail to work as they are meant to. A consistent source of glucose is required to fuel the cells. This source is achieved by digesting food and also using stored glucose within the body.

Having too much or too little glucose in our blood can ultimately jeopardise the survival of the body. Fortunately our body has a system of regulating how much glucose is present in the blood stream. The pancreas is a very important organ. Under stimulation from the central nervous system, along with releasing enzymes to aid digestion, it acts as a monitoring device for blood glucose. When you digest food, the level of glucose will inevitably rise. How much the level will rise will depend on how much sugar is contained in the food you have eaten. As too much glucose in the blood stream is a problem, the pancreas senses this and releases the hormone called insulin.

The hormone insulin signals the liver and other body cells to take glucose from the blood stream and store it to avoid damage to the body. This behaviour of stimulating cells in the body to store glucose is the reason why you gain weight. Once the liver has stored as much glucose as it can, the body begins to manufacture fat cells, which are droplets of fat contained in tissue around the body. The more glucose removed from the blood stream leads to more 'fat' cells being produced, and more 'weight' being gained. Once the level of glucose in the blood is in a desirable range the stimulus for insulin diminishes.

As has already been discussed, the 'satiety' or 'satisfaction' hormone Leptin is released when the body has received enough glucose/food. This is coupled with the feeling of being 'full'. We have all felt this feeling, and it is because there is a delay between food entering the stomach and the body realising it has had enough glucose. Whatever you consume will be digested, as long as the digestive system can handle what is being processed it will convert food into glucose. A popular reason for over-eating and gaining weight is because our behaviours over-ride the feeling of satisfaction and consumption continues. We will discuss this further when we talk about your psychology later in the book.

At some point after eating, your body will have used up the glucose/energy provided by the food and the level of glucose in your blood will fall. In this scenario, the cells within the body are not receiving enough fuel to function properly and action must be taken. The pancreas once again senses this problem and in this situation releases the hormone glucagon. Glucagon stimulates the release of stored glucose in the body. The glucose is released into the blood stream to continue to fuel the cells in the body and maintain life.

In the first stages, the required glucose will come from the liver, and once this store is depleted, the body will then begin to use the glucose stored in fat cells. At the same time as this is happening, other hormones are being released in the body to stimulate the brain to find food to supply more glucose. Similar to insulin, once the level of blood glucose is in a desirable range the stimulus for glucagon diminishes. You may remember that this stored glucose was actually the product of too much glucose in the blood at an earlier time. The ability to store energy is one of the main reasons a human being can survive for two weeks without food.

The central nervous system and the pancreas are continuously monitoring the level of blood glucose and releasing hormones to stimulate either the removal or addition of glucose to the blood stream. Their aim is to keep the level of glucose within a desirable range where the cells are receiving just enough fuel to function. It is an action performed by the body automatically and our only influence on it is the food we eat and when we eat.

Another source of glucose can be found stored in muscle. Muscle is everywhere in your body and not restricted to the ones we can see on the outside of our bodies. Some of our most important muscles are those around our heart that going on working our whole lives with no real input from ourselves apart from giving them the energy they need to keep working.

Muscle needs more energy to maintain itself compared to fat, which means your metabolism is much higher. The greater muscle mass you have, the greater amounts of glucose are required. Imagine two people, but one person had more muscle mass compared to the other. If the two ate the same meal, the person with less muscle is likely to store more glucose as fat. The reason being is that when the glucose from the food enters the blood stream the person with more muscle demands more glucose to fuel the cells in these tissues.

Without as much muscle, the glucose is stored in greater amounts as fat. This is the reason why it is recommended to build muscle as a part of your exercise regime. Muscle does a very good job of burning calories (energy) and therefore less glucose gets stored than if the muscle was not present.

The behaviour of using stored glucose in fat cells clearly highlights how physical weight is lost. The biggest challenge is to lose fat without losing muscle. As you have learnt muscle does a great job of solving the problem of too much glucose/food consumed. My recommendation is to begin to introduce weight or strength training into your exercise routine. This is not about becoming a weight lifter; this is about working the muscles so that they require more energy to work.

If you are ever in a little discomfort the day after weight based exercise, or actually any exercise, take heart that this pain means the body is using up more glucose and energy to heal its muscles. This is a good thing as the body will be more likely to take glucose stored as fat rather than remove glucose from the very thing it is aiming to repair. As a result of all of this, weight may be lost in the process, even the day after exercise. In the next chapter, when we discuss starvation you will learn that losing weight quickly leads to losing muscle as the body fears for its survival.

I have already briefly discussed metabolism, but I feel it is important to understand it a little more as the word is thrown about a lot with regards to weight loss. Metabolism can be explained in many ways and often is. It is referred to as the process of turning food/glucose into energy our cells can use. Many people take ownership of their metabolism and its characteristics, by say theirs is high or low. In simple terms metabolism is the amount of energy (calories) the body requires maintaining itself. The energy source primarily comes from glucose transported around the body by the blood stream. Everything happening in your body demands energy from keeping our blood warm to making the smallest muscles in our eyes move.

Metabolism is very important concept with regards to weight loss as it has a significant impact on how the body behaves. Let us once again return to the big picture of what the body does. As we have discussed the highest priority is to survive. The behaviour that sums up our survival is the ability to adapt. Metabolism is a specific behaviour, which helps your body to adapt to its immediate environment at any moment in time.

The recommended daily allowance of calories, posted on food labels is directly related to your metabolism. The value of about 2000 calories, depending on whether you are male or female is what scientists have recommended as the amount of glucose required to fuel the average body for activities in an average 24-hour period. The problem comes when you try to describe the average body and an average 24 hours.

Top Olympic swimmers can consume up to 12000 calories a day while training, but they do not store this glucose as fat, because their metabolism is continuously burning this potential energy. Likewise if you are sitting down all day, you are still using energy to maintain the cells of the body, but the demand for energy and associated glucose is a lot less. I mentioned in my previous example that muscle can be important to weight loss. Muscle requires more energy and glucose to maintain itself even if it is not always being used. All of this information supports the importance of burning calories through movement and exercise and the overall balance of energy or potential energy (glucose) within the body.

Your metabolism will be most active first thing in the morning, as your body has been without glucose for a long period of time. Your metabolism's 'speed' or 'activity' will depend on the physical activities you do, but in general become less active throughout the day. The lowest amount of activity is while you are asleep. This is why late night food and snacks are not advised because the glucose is not required by the body, and is therefore stored. The advice of eating like a king at breakfast, a prince at lunch and a pauper in the evening relates to the concept of when your metabolism for normal functioning is most active and requires potential energy.

I began this chapter by discussing how your surroundings will inevitable effect the digestive system, particularly if the body is in danger, under threat, or suffering from stress. Efforts are taken away from the system to concentrate on more immediate areas of the body. It would be beneficial if you were never scared, or engaged in anything that may stimulate the fight-or-flight response, but this is a lot easier said than done. We will discuss this aspect further when we discuss your psychology with respect to why you are individual. It is something we can have some control over and do something about.

Similar to the pancreas continuously monitoring the level of blood glucose, and taking action, the central nervous system is also monitoring our surroundings and it not as clear-cut to say whether the fight-or-flight or the rest-and-digest responses are in action. They are a balance and can change at any time to suit your surroundings. It is no wonder that people get digestive complaints due to stress. Being in a heightened attentive state can cause the digestive system to be neglected.

Another big problem with stress and perceived danger is that the body is primed for action and as a result the adrenal glands release the hormone cortisol. Cortisol stimulates the body to increase blood sugar because it expects the body to either fight or run, which obviously requires a great deal of energy. The body has already pre-empted this need for energy and has a ready source available.

Hundreds of years ago, our threat to survival may have been dangerous animals, which we would have either fought or run from, using up this blood glucose. In today's world, a photocopier breaking or a traffic jam can trigger your stress response. The release of cortisol and a rise in blood glucose occurs but by sitting in an office or car, does not use it up. As has been discussed, heightened levels of glucose in the blood stream can cause problems for any amount of time. The body will then store this glucose possibly as fat, obviously causing a weight gain.

It is not a coincidence that you 'crave' certain foods. If our central nervous system perceives danger, although efforts are drawn away from the digestive system, you still require glucose for fight or flight. The central nervous system has the ability to coordinate your senses (sight, hearing, touch, taste and smell) and limbs to seek out high in glucose/sugar foods. This can explain why we desire certain foods at certain times.

CHAPTER 4

STARVATION

In chapter 1, I mentioned that one of the easiest ways to get weight loss results was to cut down on the potential energy (glucose) going into the body. I still believe this is true, but due to your highest priority being survival and body's ability to adapt, it is worth discussing what happens when your intake of food is reduced.

The most extreme way of losing weight is to starve yourself of food. It does not matter who you are, over a long period of time without food you will lose weight. A big problem occurs when food is reintroduced at any point in the process of starvation. Starvation can cause long-term damage to the body and will eventually lead to death. The process of starvation is a perfect illustration of your innate ability to survive. Research shows that an average human being can survive up to two weeks without food. The exact time does depend on the environment someone is in and their physical make up, but in this example let us look at the process. The following example is not a step-by-step account of what happens in the process of starvation, but will help you appreciate what is involved. Once we have looked at what happens, we can discuss why it is important to understand with regards to weight loss.

Hunger is the first tell tale sign your body is requesting food and energy. As time passes your stomach will go from making inauspicious audible sounds to causing you painful cramps. You will feel weak and lethargic, light headed and disorientated. You will lose fat and muscle from your body, and as a result becoming thinner and weaker the longer you go without food. Your major organs and in particular your heart will fail to function and as a result you will die.

What we see, feel and experience throughout starvation are the consequences of what the body is doing to keep itself alive. The majority of physical behaviours happen with no conscious thought or input from yourself. Because the process of starvation happens over a period of time, this example also demonstrates what parts of the body are most important for survival. The reason for death maybe described as starvation, but the actual cause is often the breakdown of muscle tissue in the body, which eventually triggers lethal heart failure. But what is actually happening inside the body?

From the beginning, your body is giving you conscious signs that it needs food, the first being hunger. Hunger is not easily defined but can only be described as a longing for food. A hormone called Ghrelin causes the longing you feel and is released from the walls of the stomach and small intestine into the bloodstream. The result of the hormone being released gives you the feeling of hunger and stimulates your central nervous system to find food.

The audible sounds we hear are often referred to as 'growling' or 'rumbling', and can be experienced whether digestion of food is happening or not. It is probably easier to start by talking about what happens when food is passing through the body and then discuss why the noises are still heard when there is no food present. The sounds are primarily due to how food moves through your digestive system.

Stimulated by the central nervous system, waves of <u>muscle</u> contractions starting in the stomach move and push the contents continually downward in a process called peristalsis. In addition to moving your meal along its digestive path, these contractions also help churn food, liquid and different digestive juices together, rendering them into a gooey mixture known as chyme. The noises we hear are the result of this process. Along with the food and liquid chyme, gases and air are also present. As all these ingredients get pushed around and broken down into easy-to-absorb bits, pockets of air and gas also get squeezed and create the noises we hear.

If your stomach is empty, the muscle contractions and noises will still occur. The reason has to do with hunger and appetite. About two hours after your stomach empties itself, it begins to produce hormones that stimulate local nerves to send a message to the brain. The brain replies by signalling for the digestive muscles to restart the process of peristalsis. Two results occur: First, the contractions sweep up any remaining food that was missed the first time around. Second, the vibrations of an empty stomach make you hungry.

Feeling lethargic, light-headed and disorientated is the consequence of low levels of blood glucose, which was discussed at length in chapter 3. If the brain is not receiving enough glucose it will lead to the problems listed above and in worse cases lead to weakness, passing out or fainting. Fainting is an important survival behaviour itself and occurs when the body has sensed the brain is lacking glucose to function properly. In an effort to get more blood/glucose to the brain, the body initiates a behaviour where the brain can get closer to the level of the heart and therefore is not working as hard pumping blood against gravity. The body will collapse in one swift motion and shows how the body is able to adapt to a situation quickly and focus its efforts on what is most important. In this example, what was most important was getting more glucose to the brain, which coordinates the actions of the whole body.

We have talked at length about the role of blood glucose and it is worth mentioning again with regards to starvation. By not eating, you are starving the body of glucose, and therefore energy. When glucose is not coming from a regular outside source (food), action must be taken. As we have discussed in the previous chapter, the central nervous system can stimulate the pancreas to release the hormone glucagon, to stimulate the liver and other cells of the body to release their stored glucose. Losing the glucose stored within the liver is an everyday occurrence and is expected. Losing glucose stored in fat and muscle can lead to problems.

Excessive fat can be lost without concern, but it is beneficial in small amounts as it serves as protection to internal organs and systems. It also serves as insulation to help keep the body warm enough. Losing glucose stored in muscle can lead to long lasting damage and ultimately be fatal. The body contains three types of muscle tissue, skeletal muscle, smooth muscle and cardiac muscle. They have significant differences, but at the same time are all made up of cells, and as you know, cells need energy to function. If the glucose in muscle is not replenished the tissue will eventually break down often referred to as muscle wastage.

In times of starvation the body is concentrating its efforts on the most important functions. Skeletal muscle is usually lost first. Although this type of muscle helps us fight or run from danger, what is more important is keeping the body functioning. Smooth muscle, which is involved in digestion, is lost next. The body concludes that food is not on its way, and therefore decides to sacrifice the energy stored in this muscle to fuel most important type of muscle that keeps your heart beating; cardiac muscle.

Up to the point of death the body will sacrifice other muscles and tissues in an attempt to keep the heart beating. Energy is continuously being directed towards the most vital areas of the body, but at the same time avoiding as much damage to itself as possible. Heart failure happens because the cardiac muscle which contracts to make the heart pump blood around the body fails to function. In other words this imperative muscle has run out of energy and life can no longer be sustained.

This example of how the body behaves with regards to starvation certainly confirms it does whatever in can to sustain life for as long as it can. The ability to adapt is also highlighted by a number of automatic behaviours. The body directs its efforts and energy to those cells, parts and systems, which are most important for survival. It shows that the body has the ability to store energy, so in times of famine, it can survive for a certain period time until food is attainable. Most importantly it highlights our ability to adapt to our immediate environment, which is the main reason why we are so successful at survival.

Throughout the process of starvation the central nervous system is assessing what is going on inside and outside of the body. Although the body requires glucose, the brain is conscious that glucose may not be coming and begins to adapt by slowing your metabolism, as was discussed in the previous chapter. The thyroid gland, which regulates metabolism will also adjust your inside body temperature, so less glucose/energy is being used up in a bid to prolong life.

Let us return to the big picture of how your body behaves with regards to gaining, maintaining and losing weight. I'm sure you have heard of the term 'crash-diet'. A crash diet is consciously starving the body of food in the hope weight/fat will be lost. As is observed in the stages of starvation, after a specific period of time the body will begin to use up fat/energy stored in tissue, and as a result 'weight' will be lost. At the same time energy stored in muscle may also be used to fuel the body. The biggest problem of crash dieting is that it cannot be sustained for any length of time without real conscious effort. The longer the body goes without an outside source of glucose the more physical pain is felt.

To take the feelings of hunger and physical pain away, the answer is to eat. If food is available, it becomes a psychological challenge to resist eating food and in most cases cannot be denied. The experience of pain anywhere in the body is a sign that action needs taking, which can be seen as another survival behaviour.

It is important to realize what happens when an outside source of glucose becomes available at any point during starvation. In the early stages when blood glucose becomes low, the pancreas releases the hormone glucagon and the liver uses its store of energy to raise the level of blood glucose. At the same time hormones released within the body are signalling that food is required. If food is consumed, the pancreas will now begin to release the hormone insulin if blood glucose rises. The liver replenishes its store of glucose, and any surplus is stored in adipose tissue as fat. Your body is always releasing insulin or glucagon to keep the balance of blood glucose within a desired range to sustain life.

Once the body has begun the process of using glucose stored as fat and in muscles, the reaction to an outside source of glucose can be slightly different. A consequence of crash diets is that when the body finally consumes food, extra fat/weight will be gained. The body is demanding glucose and lots of it, the hunger hormones are intense and you will probably eat a large amount of food in a short amount of time. Your blood stream will be inundated with glucose and causes the body to take drastic action. Glucose is stored and weight is regained.

Another reason for extra weight gain is that when the body is reintroduced to food, the central nervous system may be on alert that starvation could happen again. In this case, the body will keep your metabolism low, and store energy for if starvation and the threat to survival reoccur. Once again this shows how the body is able to adapt to its surroundings and keep you alive.

If your consumption of calories in a 24-hour period is reduced it must be done so in small increments, so as not to alarm the central nervous system into thinking the body is in danger of starvation. Another piece of advice often heard is to eat 'little and often'. This is the same principle as what we have just discussed. If the same amount of food was eaten in smaller amounts or over a longer period of time, the body is able to create a balance. This means the glucose in the blood is more stable; less energy is stored and is therefore used primarily as fuel for the cells of the body.

It is worth discussing a serious health problem related to weight gain and why it happens. Type 2 diabetes is the chronic result of too much glucose in the blood. Too much glucose in the blood damages blood vessels themselves and leads to a number of serious problems including heart and kidney failure and ultimately death if not treated. Normally the pancreas, through the release of the hormone insulin would stimulate the body to remove glucose from the blood stream. Diabetes is a condition where the pancreas fails to produce enough of the hormone, or the insulin produced does not work properly.

Type 2 diabetes is the consequence of the pancreas not being able to adapt to demands placed upon it and as a result does not function properly. Losing weight and eating a low-sugar diet can help keep blood glucose at a desirable level. In worse cases where the pancreas fails to work at all, insulin must be injected into the body. Throughout this book we have discussed the importance of the body being able to adapt in order to survive. Diabetes shows that when the ability to adapt is jeopardised, overall survival is threatened.

To conclude, crash diets and denying the body of food are not suitable ways to lose weight. The body is able to adapt to the lack of glucose from an outside source. The problem comes when food is re-introduced to the body causing the behaviours we have discussed. The likelihood of regaining weight is high, and in times of famine, tissues including muscles can be permanently affected. Keeping your metabolism stable, by eating suitable foods is a very important aspect of weight loss. Weight loss can be achieved by balancing your energy requirements with the potential energy you consume. Reducing calorie consumption must be done in small increments so as not alarm the central nervous system that starvation and a threat to survival may occur.

CHAPTER 5

EATING BEHAVIOURS

At the beginning of this book I stated that many people know what they have to do to lose weight, but the challenge is to put their knowledge into action. This may be the position you are in, or have been for some time. I also discussed that to be able to put knowledge into action; you must first have the correct information, and also understand how you and your body behave. Up to this point we have discussed at length the most important aspects of how your body gains, maintains and loses weight physically. Keeping in mind that our highest priority is survival, we have also discussed how our bodies behave if there is perceived danger compared to when there is not.

All the physical parts, systems and behaviours of the body achieve survival by adapting to whatever is happening at any given time. This can range from the amount of glucose in the blood stream to bodily reflexes that avoid danger which are on the outside of the body. Every behaviour is processed by your central nervous system made up of your brain and spinal cord. This system stimulates parts of the body and monitors the results to achieve a balance and homeostasis within the body so life can be sustained.

Food has many purposes in our society beyond the satisfaction of hunger and the need to maintain life. Eating food is a very social thing to do. There are certain activities that are associated with food, like eating out with friends or going to the cinema and eating popcorn. Food festivals are popular as are reading about cookery, and watching it on television programmes. If these activities and the associated consumption of food is done in moderation, then continue to enjoy. There are however behaviours related to food, which are unsuitable and can jeopardise weight loss success. Food is often seen as a comfort when someone feels unhappy or bored. It is used to tranquillise whatever feelings are being felt. You can also crave certain kinds of foods depending on what the body requires. In a psychological sense, chocolate contains chemicals, which can enhance your mood and cause the brain to release more 'feel good' hormones.

From this point on in the book, it is even more important to read the information in relation to yourself. We have obviously looked at many aspects of the human body, but will now be looking at behaviours that are specific to you.

We all function in a very similar way physically, but what sets us apart and makes us unique is our psychology. At this point I would like to ask you a very important question. The answer will help you get the best out of this book with regards to your own situation.

What has stopped you up to now from achieving your goal of losing weight?

Please take some time to think about this question, and trust whatever comes to your mind first is the truth. Your answer to this question will be unique to you. I cannot address your specific answer in this book, but we will be discussing some familiar topics and later looking at how we can resolve what has stopped you up to now achieving weight loss success.

From reading the previous chapters, you have probably come to realise that many of the physical behaviours within the body are automatic, and unfortunately we have no control of them. What we do have control over is providing the body with the correct type and amount of food. A big problem with losing weight is the behaviour of over-eating. If you are already on a healthy eating or weight loss programme, your problem may be that you occasionally lose motivation. You may fall into bad habits of snacking on unsuitable foods or not monitoring the calories you are consuming.

These are behaviours that you may want to change because they do not support your weight loss. Recognise your unique behaviours now, and try to be as specific as possible. You may snack on chocolate, but start to think about when you snack? What time of day? What is happening around you at the time you snack? These answers are all unique to you.

Before we move on, let us return to why and how we gain weight physically. The body must be given enough calories for it to function in its daily activities. In simple terms, weight gain is due to the body receiving more calories than are used by the body and these are subsequently stored as fat. As was discussed early in this book the consumption of food has the biggest impact on weight, and over-eating jeopardises your weight loss success.

We have discussed in past chapters that the 'satisfaction' hormone leptin is released in the body to stimulate the central nervous system to cease food consumption. There is often a delay in the hormone having an effect on our central nervous system and food may already be in the digestive tract before we feel the body has had enough. This delay could be the reason why weight is gained, as we do not get a 'sign' that we have had 'enough' food and glucose until it is too late. You also experience cravings for a certain kinds of food depending on what the body requires. Repeated over-eating or snacking on high in glucose food in this manor can obviously cause weight gain if the body is not using the calories it is consuming. Another physical reason for over-eating is that hunger can be confused with thirst. Do you really know the difference between the body requesting food, or just water? If you do feel hungry outside of meal times, I recommend that you drink water. This action can fill the stomach and can take away the feeling of hunger that you may have.

Although there are many physical reasons why you may over-eat. I believe the real reasons are associated with your psychology. Many people watch what they eat, read the magazines, but lose motivation and succumb to eating unsuitable foods. Many people are on a constant merry-go-round of dieting. They get focused, do everything correct, something happens, motivation is lost and they have to start again. You may be in a similar situation where you may be very good at making a decision to stick to a diet, or weight loss programme but struggle to follow it at all times. People who do have weight loss success achieve it by sticking to whatever diet or plan they are following.

Slimming magazines are full of stories and photographs of people achieving weight loss success. These stories and photographs may be a motivation to you, and spur you on to keep going, but the truth is there situation is as unique as yours.

The reason why they gained weight and behave the way they do towards food and exercise will be completely different to you. When the real reasons are addressed and resolved this can clear the way to introduce more beneficial behaviours and be in control of them. This commitment and motivation towards what you want is what we are now going to discuss with regards to your psychology.

When we talk about psychology, it is important to understand that it is very closely related to your physical body and in particular your central nervous system. It is also difficult to explain what the psychological 'mind' is, but we know it is related to the physical body by a very simple question. If I asked you to think of your favourite food as you read these words, or maybe even imagine biting into a lemon. Did you notice what happened? Your mouth started to salivate. There was no food or lemon? By asking you to imagine, your body was able to react to words I said.

Imagination is the realm of the mind. This is a small example of how language and imagination can affect behaviours related to your physical body. Your mind is a mixture of intellect and emotion. Emotions can be defined as strong mental feelings, and are directly related to how you experience the world. How you feel emotions is unique to you. The same stimulus to someone else could make him or her excited and you frightened or upset. Why the same stimulus makes you feel differently is based on your unique psychology and will be discussed very soon.

Your individuality has a lot to do with emotions and how you feel about certain things. Emotions are felt physically and are described perfectly comparing the act of crying and the emotion of sadness. Tear ducts around the eye release fluid to keep the eye clean and healthy. If there is a foreign object on the eye, our central nervous system will sense this and initiate the ducts to release greater amounts of fluid to flush this unwanted material out. In an emotional sense, when we feel sadness, there may be no foreign object in our eye, but the central nervous system still initiates the same behaviour.

I appreciate, up to now you may not have thought about how closely your emotions and physical behaviours are, but it happens all over the body and is primarily how you perceive your immediate surroundings.

The easiest way to describe your psychology is the 'filters through which you experience the world'. It is your beliefs, values, opinions, memories and experiences that make you so unique. No one else will have the same psychology as you. To understand how you achieved the beliefs, opinions etc... that make you so unique, we must once again refer to our highest priority: survival.

Just as the body directs its efforts towards survival, the mind will also. From the minute your central nervous system was developed inside your mother's womb, you have had the ability to sense your immediate surroundings and therefore had the ability to adapt to any scenario that may occur. You have also had the ability to remember these experiences and most importantly learn from them. This learning behaviour and the ability to remember is imperative for survival.

From the experiences you have, it informs your central nervous system what is safe and unsafe with regards to survival. We have discussed that the central nervous system is at all times monitoring what goes on inside and outside the body. We have also discussed how we are constantly in a balance of fight-or-flight or rest-and-digest response. Depending on our situation, the body is either concentrating on the short-term immediate threat to survival, or preparing and repairing itself ready for any further threat.

Up to now we have not discussed what is perceived as dangerous, or in other words what triggers our fight-or-flight response and cause our central nervous system to prepare the body for action? We already know it has something to do with our immediate surroundings, but more importantly it concerns your perception of those surroundings. Your perception of your surroundings is unique and a result of your psychology, the combination of your experiences up to now in your life.

The topic of survival has been a key point throughout this book, as it has the power to explain why we do the things we do on a physical and psychological level. We will continue this theme of survival as we discuss psychology. At this point, it is important to understand how your psychology has developed and why it makes you so unique. We can then discuss how this relates to your eating behaviours on a day-to-day basis.

At any given moment in time it is thought that there are up to two million possible bits of information your senses (sight, hearing, touch, taste and smell) have the ability to recognise. As you read this, you may not be conscious of it all, but all of your senses are active, you are using your eyes, you may hear sounds and feel the ground beneath your feet. Often we only notice something when it could be a threat to us. An example of this is hearing a loud noise and your automatic reaction is to jump. The physical jump is a response that your mind perceives there is danger. Before you know it, you are alert and ready to take action to avoid any danger.

Like many physical actions you only see the consequences of what your physical body has accomplished. All in a split second, your central nervous system has received the information from your ears, decided what to do, and caused a reaction in your body to avert the perceived danger. The question is, what makes you jump? Not everyone will jump at a loud noise, so what makes people so different. It has everything to do with your immediate surroundings at the time and your psychology, which is constructed of your memories etc... First and foremost you must be in a position to hear the noise, and secondly it depends whether you perceive that noise as danger.

Let us return to the possible two million bits of information in our immediate surroundings. Our senses receive the information and it passes to the central nervous system. Scientists and philosophers have debated the link between the body, brain and mind for hundreds of years. This book is not going to discuss the link, but it is important to recognise there is one.

As I have demonstrated earlier in this chapter I asked you to imagine eating your favourite food or biting into a lemon. This simple question had the power of making you salivate. The easiest way to describe the difference between the brain and the mind is to say that the **brain receives information, and the mind makes sense of it.** The information may be visual (sight), auditory (sound), kinesthetic (feeling), olfactory (smell) or gustatory (taste).

If I asked you to imagine eating your least favourite food, your mouth will now probable dry up rather than salivate. In worst cases you may even feel sick at the thought of a type of food. After the mind has given meaning to the information, the central nervous system will make a decision of how to act in accordance with survival. As I have already mentioned, your psychology and mind make you unique, how you react or feel about something will be acutely different to what other people will think.

As has already been discussed briefly, your psychology started to develop from as early as when you were in your mother's womb. From an early age you are experiencing many things and hearing people's opinions and beliefs. You begin by knowing nothing about the world you live in, to believing everything that you experience and are told. You rely on your parents or guardian for survival, not only physically but also to have your emotional needs met. You learn to understand and speak your language to be able to communicate with people and the world around you.

Everyone in your life, especially your parents and those closest to you are providing you with an abundance of information. You are also likely to be taught what is safe and what is unsafe on a regular basis. This was not limited to physical safety, but also what you were allowed to do or not do to be accepted and loved by the people around you. You believe all the information as the truth.

As you continue to age, your desire is to become more independent. By the time you are in your early twenties, you are so full up of experiences, beliefs, opinions, and combinations of these, you along with most people live out the rest of their lives playing out the patterns. Every second of our life we are having experiences. Each experience and behaviour or thought about it turns into a memory, which is recorded by the mind. It is as if it is filed away as a 'learning' and can be referred to again if something else similar comes up. The filters through which we see the world are a combination of these experiences stored as memories. Patterns, behaviours and habits happen because the experiences and the outcome happen again and again over time that they reinforce their own validity.

So how does this all relate to your eating behaviours? Firstly, I want you think back to your childhood and think about how you used to eat as a family, what would you eat and how big were the portions? How does this compare to how you eat and how much you eat? Are they similar?

What was said about food when you were a child? Were you always made to finish your meal? Was there some kind of punishment if you did not? The punishment could be that you were not allowed to go out and play, or have dessert?

Was your mother or father overweight or on a diet? How did the people you know behave around food?

As I have already said, from a very early age, your brain/mind is like a sponge. Because you have nothing to compare people's opinions and beliefs to, you treat them as the truth and can carry them throughout your life acting on them automatically and unconsciously. Parents will often offer sweets and biscuits as a reward or as a comfort to falling over or disappointments. As a result some overweight adults continue to console themselves throughout their lives with excessive food.

Your parents may not have been the best role models regarding food, but unconsciously you maybe following their behaviours up to this day. This is related to the mental challenge we have discussed from the beginning of this book. The aim is to introduce new behaviours into your lifestyle, which help rather than hinder you losing weight.

The reason why you fall into bad habits is ultimately because of unconscious patterns repeating themselves over and over again. In the next chapter we will discuss changing your behaviours to achieve weight loss success.

Your eating behaviours may not necessarily be associated with something you learnt as a child to do with food. It may have something to do with a comment or opinion someone made about your appearance. Once again you have believed it as being true. When did weight become a problem? Did you start gaining weight when something significant happened in your life? Beliefs and behaviours can happen through repetition or significant emotional events that impact your life forever unless they are resolved. It could be a misunderstanding or a joke said by someone, but what is most important is how you perceived it and how it has affected your life and weight loss success.

We also cannot escape the bigger picture of what is beautiful in today's society. In some countries big is beautiful, but in others such as the UK and America, being thin seems to be the aim. The desire to feel beautiful is the aim of most people, because it has so much to do with being loved and accepted. Rejection can be perceived as a threat, so the desire is to avoid this, and find happiness.

Along with our own survival there is an innate drive to reproduce and have a piece of us survive for further generations. We consider beauty as a fundamental factor of finding a partner. Just as emotions can affect our physical body, the opposite is also true. Losing weight is as much about health as it is looking and feeling great. Is 'looking good' the number one reason why you want to lose weight?

All these examples show how important it is to recognise your beliefs, patterns and behaviours. Some of which could be a hindrance to your weight loss success. Many beliefs and behaviours were installed into your psychology at such an early age you cannot remember them. Just as the physical body has automatic actions, so does the psychological mind.

Throughout the day, many of your actions, decisions and behaviours are unconscious. There will be behaviours that you learnt when you were a child that you still use in everyday life. Even in adult life there will be activities that are new to you but eventually become unconscious and easy to do without constant conscious thought.

Driving is an excellent example of how you have learnt a skill. At some point you did not know how to drive, you began to learn and it took time to master. But after a while, it becomes 'second-nature'. This kind of scenario, but with different content has happened throughout your life and allows you to live the life you do.

Learnt behaviours such as being polite and saying 'please' and 'thank-you' are positive and help you in your social life. If however you were punished or scared to leave food on your plate, then this can be kept in your unconscious mind throughout your life and could be a reason why you still have to finish all your food. Emotional pain can be as bigger threat to the psychological mind as physical pain. If you knew that finishing your food would avoid this pain, then as a young child you would do it. A consequence of this is that you have grown up with an unconscious behaviour or belief that consuming food helps to suppress emotional pain. This may be a reason why you 'emotionally eat'.

CHAPTER 6

GOING BACK IN TIME

By writing this book, my aim is to help people get in the right frame of mind for weight loss success. I also wanted to provide some clarity about how the body gains, maintains and loses weight physically.

My hope is that you have begun to recognize how your psychology has a major impact on your weight loss and eating behaviours. It is imperative that you address the real reasons why you may over-eat, or lose motivation when you are following a weight loss programme. The real reasons are most often due to habitual patterns built from your past experiences. These experiences have formed beliefs and behaviours that you have about yourself and the world around you. It can range from how you were always told to finish whatever food was on your plate, to falling over and being consoled with sweets and chocolates. A comment may have been made about your physical appearance that has made you conscious that you will not be scene as being beautiful unless you change.

By your early twenties, you are so full up of beliefs, values and memories that you will probably play out the same behaviours, patterns and habits unless a significant emotional event changes your life drastically. A significant emotional event can cause a problem to occur, as much as go away. The behaviours are so established that you have trouble changing them as they have served you up to now with regards to survival. Consciously you want to change, but to do this you must address the unconscious side of your mind, which holds your memories.

It is very difficult to help you change your beliefs and behaviours through talking to you through a book, as it will depend on your unique situation and what experiences you have had as a young child and throughout your life with regards to weight. Changing or resolving behaviours and habits as we have discussed, is all to do with your perception of the world you live in. This perception has been built by the memories of your experiences up to this stage of your life. The memories you have can be recalled at any moment in time using your imagination. I could ask you to remember something that you ate yesterday, last week or last year and through using your psychological mind, you would be able to describe that food. You may also remember where you were, whom you were with and what time of day it was. Even though the scenario happened some time ago, your imagination is able to build an image or a collection of images now.

Your life is made up of countless experiences and as a result countless memories of what happened. These memories have been collected over the years. Many of them are useful and help you know what is safe and unsafe, and what may help you and what will not. When an experience, image or memory in your life becomes repetitive, the body and mind become accustomed to it, believing it as true.

As you go through life there are certain behaviours or habits that do not support something in our lives. This book discusses weight loss, but it could be true for any situation in your life where you require change. To address and resolve this behaviour, you must explore where and when the behaviour or habit began. Once you have recalled this memory you can determine why it started. You can also notice that it was not a problem before this time. Ultimately the aim is to change the meaning of what you experienced.

From birth, the most influential people in your early life were your parents or guardians. Along with other family and friends you will have picked up and adapted countless behaviours, beliefs, thoughts, opinions, values, mannerisms etc...

If you think about some of the behaviours you have concerning your weight and/or appearance, where did they come from? Did someone say something? When did weight become a problem?

It is so important that the root problem is addressed, and not the symptoms. It can be said that being overweight is a symptom of a problem, rather being the problem itself.

CHAPTER 7

CHANGE YOUR BEHAVIOUR

By reading this book you will have realised that losing weight has a lot more to do with your behaviour than anything else. I believe that you can achieve the weight loss you desire in a healthy way. I hope you have a better idea of how your body behaves and you can make your own choices about what food to eat. Be careful of the potential energy (glucose) you consume compared to what your body actually requires to function on a daily basis.

Exercise is an important contributor to weight loss but also for a healthy life. There are thousands of types of exercise you can do. Most importantly exercise should be enjoyable. Many people hear that a particular type of exercise is best for weight loss. Initially there will be motivation to take part in the exercise, but after a while, if it is not enjoyable the desire will fade.

What exercise do you enjoy? Whatever it is, go and enjoy it. Ignore all the tables that say how many calories you can burn in an hour doing different exercises. It is better to regularly exercise than not at all.

Many people do not know what exercise they enjoy. My recommendation to you is that you put on your favourite CD and dance. Dancing can be done anywhere and at any age. If you have children and family, get them involved also and just go for it.

The reason why you gained weight in the first place or continue to over-eat and fall into bad habits is primarily down to your psychology. Many of the reasons cannot be reached by simply talking about them, as they lie much deeper as habits and patterns, which have been reinforced by following them repetitively.

Always remember that you are built for survival in a psychological and physical sense of the word. We are able to survive because we have the ability to adapt and keep a balance and homeostasis in our lives. What you experience is always the consequence of your body and mind reacting to your surroundings.

Why we are able to survive and are on this planet? I will let you decide.

WHAT NEXT?

The team at ShippShape would love to hear your opinion of this book and whether you enjoyed it. We aim to give you the best service we can and we continually do this by responding to your feedback. We might include it on the ShippShape website, so please give us your name and contact details.

Send your opinions and your biggest learning to **david@shippshape.com**

COME TO A SHIPPSHAPE EVENT

You can come to events for people wanting to get in the right frame of mind – visit the ShippShape website for dates and venues.

SEE A MEMBER OF THE TEAM

Our commitment to you is to help you change unhelpful behaviours that jeopardise your weight loss success. Why not see a member of the ShippShape team one-to-one to get accelerated results.

www.ingramcontent.com/pod-product-compliance
Lightning Source LLC
Chambersburg PA
CBHW060643290526
45793CB00001B/377